Table of Contents

Introduction

What Is Emotional Eating?

My Own Experience: Brief bio

Chapter 1 — Emotional Eating, Wellness, and You

Chapter 2 — It's Okay to Eat Your Feelings

Chapter 3 — 5 Roadblocks Which Stop You from Connecting to Your Body, and Knowing What It Says

Chapter 4 — Take Control of Your Life: Put Shame and Guilt Behind You

Chapter 5 — HALT Framework to Stop Overeating

Understand the Difference Between Overeating and Binge Eating

Chapter 6 — Listen to Your Body Signals

Chapter 7 — Manage Internal Chaos Created by High Cortisol to Prevent Eating Emotionally

Chapter 8 — 4 Hormones Which Define Your Road to Happiness

Chapter 9 — Science Behind Habit Formation

Chapter 10 — Eating Mindfully

Chapter 11 — The Fundamentals of Nutrition

Chapter 12 — You Can Work to Your Full Potential from Today

Introduction
MY STORY
What Is Emotional Eating?

All kinds of emotions afflict you at varying times. When some emotions, situations, relationships become difficult to handle, how do you deal with it? Do you sit down with a peer group, or a set of sensible adults to discuss the aspects which you find overbearing or disturbing? Are you being borne down by the weight of expectations from your family, teachers/coaches, friends, and colleagues? Studies conducted in different parts of the world indicate that many people eat as a way to cope with stress resulting from situations beyond our control, and diverse emotions — a condition called emotional eating (EE) — eating high-carbohydrate, high-calorie foods of dubious or low nutritional value.

EE Is Not a Clearly Defined Issue Still

It is important to note that emotional eating is not a clearly defined issue even now, though it was identified as a problem besetting a major proportion of the population several decades ago. Quite often, EE gets mistaken for simple overeating or under eating. However, it has been recognized that you receive many different kinds of cues which trigger EE. Whether you are a restrained eater, or binge eat habitually; the chances are that you have indulged in emotional eating at some stage or the other. To assess how likely it is that you eat emotionally, watch your cues, and what you eat in response to those cues. There is much more to emotional eating than increasing food intake specifically when in a negative mood.

Understand What Can Trigger Emotional Eating

Stress causes certain regions of the brain to release chemicals — specifically, neuropeptide Y and opiates. These chemicals can trigger mechanisms that are similar to the cravings you get from fat and sugar. However, it is critical to note that emotional eating results from different emotional states — anger, happiness, anticipation, bereavement, jealousy, anxiety — as well as physical and mental health issues. What makes emotional eating so dangerous is that it makes us reach for food which is harmful for our health, and overall well-being. Whether we overeat, eat far less than our body's requirement, or practically stop eating — emotional eating hurts us by impacting our health negatively. Dieting lapses might occur when a person is in a positive mood, or in a negative one. Unfortunately, the body tends to store more fat when you are stressed as opposed to when you are relaxed.

What Is Your Normal Response to Stress?

Whether you are facing relationship blues, workplace challenges, grave illness in the family, have a new member of the family on the way, wondering how to raise funds to meet your commitments, or disturbed by a recent natural disaster; what is your normal response? If you are livid about some situations, or something someone has said or done; what do you do to reduce the stress? Do you hit the road for a long run, walk, or drive? Do you listen to music to calm down? Or read a book? Or do you begin to eat whatever comes to hand, especially if it is your favorite food? Many people eat when they are stressed because it distracts them.

Every Person Has Indulged in Emotional Eating at Some Stage of Life

If like many other people in the world you seek comfort from food — be it a specific kind, or just about the first thing you see — then you suffer from emotional eating (EE). Men and women are equally likely to suffer from this disorder. Unfortunately, emotional eating rarely resolves the issues which drove you to binge, but has a harmful impact on your health as you gain weight. There is nothing to be ashamed about EE. It is a disorder which can be cured without medicines, or strenuous exercise. You simply need to first accept that there is an issue, and reach out for help. The greater the proportion of negative emotions followed by food consumption, the more likely someone is to be an emotional eater.

Shocking Findings By APA

Shocking findings disclosed by a survey run by the American Psychological Association (APA) in 2013 indicated that the millennials are least geared to handling stress compared to Gen Xers and Baby Boomers. They are likeliest to give in to food cravings or eat unhealthy food; as many as 16 percent admitted to habitually skipping meals when stressed; and overeating when stressed. Similarly, women are likelier to indulge in ED than men. It could be because women are often stressed by day to day affairs, and are under intolerable pressure with regard to their weight and size.

My Own Experience

I became interested in emotional eating because from childhood food was the best way to soothe me when I was ruffled about something. It did not have to be *pakoras, halwas,* or *shahi paneer.* Often, my mother would hand me a humble samosa when she saw I was cranky, and it was adequate to cheer me up. I loved visiting the gurudwara where you would get delicious *kadha prasad* dripping with ghee and loaded with sugar. Unfortunately, it never occurred to me that eating was my reaction to stress.

Net result was that even in adulthood, if there was a complicated case among my patients, my children had exams on, especially before their board and university exams, I would allay my anxiety by reaching out for chocolates, pastries, and similar delicious, but extremely harmful foods. The impact on my body weight was disastrous, creating health issues to complicate matters further. Eventually, I began working on how to release myself from the habit of eating emotionally.

I Work to Help People Enjoy Better Health

Let me introduce myself. I am a functional medicine expert, self-made entrepreneur, mentor, and leadership coach for physicians. I use a holistic approach to help people enjoy better health by working on the causes rather than symptoms. An alumni of a renowned medical college in Amritsar, I also hold a Fellowship in Functional Medicine from American Academy of Anti-aging Medicine. Additionally, I earned an MBA in Finance from the prestigious Indian Institute of Management, Lucknow to complement my existing skills.

Even I Have a Constant Need for Pep Talk

Despite having worked at various organizations, managed large teams, having been a part of the team at Assocham to make school health guidelines, and a part of the key team of NCERT board to create a diagnostic tool for mental health diseases, when it came to food I always lost it to emotional eating. My genetic test showed that I had no satiety gene. This always made me talk to myself — talk to the negative one saying "Priti you cannot do this. You are a loser" — little realizing that such an approach was self-defeating. I would have to give myself pep talks to go ahead and achieve what I wanted to. In the long run this self-encouragement worked wonders.

The Greatest Revelation of My Life

When I realized the WHY of my problem with eating, I started working on it. The more control I had on my eating, the better my self-talk started to become. This was the greatest revelation of my life which helped me achieve lots of success and happiness thereafter. From being a textbook diabetic and obese myself, I was determined to reverse my diabetic condition, and lost 23 kilograms using my self-created "Cyclic Keto" program.

Medi-Skool was started with only one mission — to reverse chronic diabetes, obesity, and mental health issues in India. Many clients have benefitted from it so far. I hope to bring about a significant change in the lives of people by drawing upon my wealth of experience across different delivery models.

Become Smarter, Sharper, and Healthier Than Before

I have utilized my 27 years of experience in the healthcare industry to help people reverse diabetes, conquer cravings, and lose weight without going hungry. When people use the tools I have designed, it helps them become smarter, sharper, and healthier than before. My other areas of interest include gut health such as infections, allergies, irritable bowel syndrome (IBS), and hormonal imbalance such as PCOD, menopause, fibroids, mood disorders, and fatigue.

My mission is to help doctors find how to provide consistently excellent care to patients and still have the satisfying personal relationships they desire by drawing on my analytical decision-making abilities and strategic skills. I strongly believe that "a nation is as healthy as its people are".

I am right here to help you identify why, where, and when you need to eat emotionally. Then we can work together to identify your stressors, and develop a plan to help you get out of it. The impact on your health will be incalculable.

Takeaways

- ➤ Emotional Eating Is Not a Clearly Defined Issue Still
- ➤ Every Person Has Indulged In Emotional Eating at Some Stage of Life
- ➤ Watch Out for the Cues
- ➤ Even I Have a Constant Need for Pep Talk
- ➤ Become Smarter, Sharper, and Healthier Than Before

Chapter 1 — Emotional Eating, Wellness, and You

"Sugar is 20 times more addictive than cocaine." — Priti Nanda Sibal

Delving into comfort food like chocolates, candies, cookies, pizzas, burgers, ice creams, diverse sweets, potato chips, and washing it down with tea or coffee when one is struggling with emotions happens more often than most people realize. A critical question asked by many people is: why would someone want to eat when distressed, or stressed?

Filling the Void

There is an unpredictability about life about which we can do precious little. If eating comfort food every time you are stressed, over tired, ill, or simply dispirited, think of how much weight you will put on. Soon, you will begin to feel that weight has fallen in love with you, and refuses to be part away from you. In a literal sense food fills that emptiness to convey a notion of fullness, or of being complete. You want to be a person, not a shell — or at least seem so. The strange thing is that taste recognition has been found to be sharper when you eat in a happy, or otherwise positive mood. Consider the number of times you might have been unsure whether a person you know is hungry or plain cuckoo.

Four Reasons for Emotional Eating

If instead of reaching out to your own emotional support system when you are stressed, you reach for food, you set in a perennial cycle of emotional eating.

1) There is also the matter of people *not being aware* of the difference between physical hunger, and emotional hunger. The latter might be sparked by loneliness, boredom, or anger. Drinking several cups of tea or coffee because you are anxious; downing peg after peg of alcohol; all those packets of popcorns, and salted stuff don't nourish you but definitely ruin your health over the years.

2) When faced with stress and/or physical danger, the cortisol level in your body rises. It makes you crave sugar, which is one major reason why most comfort foodstuffs are sugary. It is noteworthy, that the hunger, or more accurately, eating related peptide ghrelin levels do not decline after food intake in emotional eaters, though tests have indicated that the baseline ghrelin levels are lower in emotional eaters compared to normal eaters. However, women who are anticipating some stressful situation display higher levels of ghrelin in their blood. Ghrelin profiles tend to be similar in emotional eaters, binge eaters, and obese people.

3) Major life events involving you and a loved one — weddings, childbirth, health issues, bereavement, especially bereavement which involves the death of a parent, sibling, spouse, offspring — might, and do, spark episodes of emotional eating.

4) If you indulge in negative self-talk, such as blaming yourself for a lack of will power, considering yourself "bad", or greedy; that will also set in motion further emotional eating to allay your sadness, and sense of helplessness.

Understand the Difference Between Physical Hunger and the Emotional Need to Eat

Physical Hunger

- ❖ It develops slowly over time.
- ❖ You desire a variety of food groups.
- ❖ You feel a sense of fullness, and take it as a cue to stop eating.
- ❖ You have no negative feelings about eating.

Emotional Hunger

- ❖ It comes about suddenly or abruptly.
- ❖ You crave only certain foods.

- You may binge on food, and not feel a sensation of fullness.
- You feel guilt or shame about eating.

Eat CRAP, and Become Crap

The most harmful foods you could possibly have are represented by the acronym CRAP.

C – Carbonated drinks

R – Refined sugars

A – Artificial food (As Alfred E. Newman said, "We are living in a world today where lemonade is made from artificial flavors and furniture polish is made from real lemons.")

P – Processed food

Do You Delve Into Food, or Find Some Alternative?

Delineate your normal stress response such as binge eating, or simply reaching for comfort food whether or not you are hungry before you begin to look for solutions. Once you understand the triggers, and what stresses you, stress management becomes easier because your plan will be tailor made for your needs. You need to hone your stress management skills to be able to apply your stress management plan when you notice that the stressors are triggering the desire to eat. You should be able to tell yourself, "Avoid that temptation because that's what got you to this point in the first place."

Your Wellness Is Definitely In Your Hands

Emotional eating can sabotage your mental health and your weight-loss efforts. It often leads to eating too much — especially too much of high-calorie, sweet, and fatty foods. The good news is that if you're prone to emotional eating, you can take steps to regain control of your eating habits, and get back on track with your weight-loss goals. Take a conscious decision that you want to be healthy, rather than disease ridden. Therefore, next time instead of reaching for food to serve as a distraction, reach for a phone to speak to a close friend, your mother, or siblings. Reach for a book. Switch on the music system, and groove to your favorite music. Watch some comedy shows, or films.

Takeaways

- ➢ Emotional eating is about filling a void
- ➢ Four reasons for emotional eating

- Understand the difference between physical hunger and the emotional need to eat
- Eat CRAP, and become crap
- Understand ED triggers, and what stresses you
- Your wellness is definitely in your hands

Chapter 2 — It's Okay to Eat Your Feelings

"After a good dinner, one can forgive anybody, even one's own relations."
— Oscar Wilde

You can't live a full life on an empty stomach. We need to recognize that food is a part of our lives that will never go away — we HAVE to eat every day. So, why not ENJOY it, and use food as a way to bond, connect, and celebrate with our own selves its taste and texture, instead of demonizing it as something bad, and spending our time obsessing over?

Favorite Foods Which Often Become Comfort Food

Let's do a visualization exercise. Consider what your favorite comfort food is, and try to recall where and when you first ate it. It could be anything from *kadha prasad* to ice cream, *dum biriyani*, chocolates, kebabs, *dosas*, French fries, and pizzas to steaming hot rice drenched in ghee with mashed potatoes. Typically, you will have many associations with food. It could be the place you first ate it, the occasion, the people with whom you first ate it. Even when we want to celebrate some personal milestones or happy events it usually leads to binge eating — alone, with family, friends, or colleagues.

Emotional Response to Food

When somebody has truly angered you while you were cooking, haven't you added some extra chilies in reaction? Especially, if the person annoying you is the one who is going to eat it; then, your revenge is complete. Similarly, people sometimes tear into food as though that is the enemy to be demolished, or to distract themselves when they are under severe stress. Unfortunately, every time you react that way, you only serve to hurt yourself.

Do You Eat Your Way Out of Depression?

Perhaps, the fashion industry and the entertainment industry more than the healthcare system has been responsible for developing unrealistic norms of what the ideal body image should be. Eat what you want to, and when you want to. Do you find yourself thinking wistfully, "I want someone to look at me the way I look at a chocolate cake"? When you learn to be comfortable with your own body image, that wistfulness will automatically disappear. It is the forbidden fruit that always seems sweeter, and more luscious.

Negative or Positive — Feelings Often Get Expressed Through Food

We have stopped reflecting on the feelings food evokes in us, and that is where we get derailed. We tend to forget that food is meant to be partaken to nourish us, for sustenance. Instead, it becomes a peg on which to hang emotions. The concept of emotional eating is more complicated than it is often thought to be. Overeating, uncontrolled eating, and cue-reactive eating are all reflective of ED. Let's look at these aspects below, and understand ourselves better:

Reflect on the Positive Emotions Associated with Comfort Food

Make a list of all the positive emotions and thoughts you have surrounding your comfort food. Ask yourself: what are the pleasurable ideas and feelings surrounding your favorite food, so that it has become your comfort food? How do you feel while eating it? What are your feelings before you eat it? Do you have a sense of longing, a degree of expectation? How do you feel when you are eating it? Do you enjoy a sense of satiety after you have eaten? Do you feel happier after you have eaten than you felt before you reached for your favorite food? While eating, do you experience a sense of appreciation, love, gratitude, kindness, compassion, and/or forgiveness — for yourself and for others?

List Negative Feelings Before and After Eating Comfort Food

What makes you reach for comfort food in the first place? Are you feeling unloved or alienated from family and friends? Do you retreat from the very social and emotional support you need in a crisis? Have you suffered a major bereavement or other personal loss recently? Are you trying to deal with a financial crisis? Is it because you are angry with someone, a set of people, a recent incident, or your current circumstances? Is it boredom, or loneliness? Are you feeling frustrated with how your professional or personal life is shaping up, or with the system or the establishment? Is there a sense of deprivation? Are you beset with anxiety? A sense of hurt after someone made fun of you, the way you look or dress, or your dreams and aspirations could drive you to binge on your favorite food. What about how you feel afterwards? Do you experience guilt, shame, regret, or even anger with yourself when you have indulged in comfort food? The greater the proportion of negative emotions followed by food consumption, the more likely someone is to be an emotional eater.

Change the Loop You Get into After Eating

It is more important to express your feelings, rather than suppressing them. Unfortunately, the word positive has acquired unfortunate connotations in these corona times. Still, you need to be happy, optimistic, forward-looking, and joyful. As somebody said, "Whenever I feel sad, I go to my happy place — the fridge." That is not alright as it makes you go on a guilt trip immediately after that, and undergo sufficient exercise to compensate. Try other ways to get to your happy place such as reaching out to a friend, taking a shy at some artistic venture, dancing, or taking a walk. Every time you go on an eating binge, stop to consider what triggered it and deal with it accordingly. Remember, simply knowing how that food will make you feel can change the loop you get into after eating.

The Zombie Effect

Inability to sleep, and fewer hours of sleep interrupts your circadian cycle leaving you sleep deprived, and slightly disoriented, setting off a vicious circle of extreme sense of fatigue and energy boosters. Work pressures, especially the need to meet targets, social networking online, relaxing in front of the TV, and reading books etc. online have made it more difficult for people to go to sleep, or even have sufficient time on hand to sleep adequately. To offset that fatigue, you need to have more energy boosters by way of caffeine, sugar, alcohol, and simple carbohydrates. However, these things make you drowsier. The later at night that you work, the greater are your chances of snacking unhealthily.

Takeaways

- Emotional response to food: Do you eat your way out of depression?
- Negative or positive — feelings often get expressed through food
- Reflect on the positive emotions associated with comfort food
- List negative feelings before and after eating comfort food
- Change the loop you get into after eating

Chapter 3 — 5 Roadblocks Which Stop You from Connecting to Your Body, and Knowing What It Says

"Everything I love is either illegal, immoral, or fattening."
— Ambrose Bierce

For many people, it is the last which is most troublesome. This is the 21st century, yet the shape of you is more important than how kind you are, how caring, how competent, or even how learned you are. The bane of modern living is that you are expected to conform to some highly impractical shape and size, regardless of whether the kind of work you do — at home or office — supports or justifies that kind of body form. The irony is that your size is less important than your own body image. Also, think of societal expectations which create roadblocks in the path of connecting with our bodies.

Our Feelings Often Get Intricately Interwoven With Food

Some of these feelings tend to be influenced by our earliest experiences. How often have you seen that when a little one is bawling, a family elder advises a new mother to feed the baby without even trying to check what could be the baby's distress? For all you know, the baby might just want some rocking to soothe her, or might need to sleep. It inculcates a lifelong association between food and relief from distress, which lays the foundation of eating to allay feelings of sadness, anxiety, even anger. Researchers have found that the co-occurrence of specific feelings and food intake lies at the root of many eating disorders.

I) When Feeding Becomes the Panacea for All Ills

Childhood lays the foundation for emotional eating in later years. When a toddler is just learning to walk (and some kids learn at even eight months!), it is perfectly normal for a few knocks against furniture, tripping over the carpet or exposed wiring, even rolling down the slope of the main gate — as long as there are no fractures or major abrasions. While you should pick up your little sweetheart, and comfort her; you shouldn't offer her the bottle or the breast unless she is hungry.

Comfort Food Is Necessary Even in Growing Up Years

Somehow, we associate eating comfort food as something you do when you are getting on in years. That is not so. So, if your adolescent child wants some ice cream or chocolate to deal with losing a match, not performing as well as expected during a concert or a championship, or doing badly at an exam; that is alright. Look at the bright side of it — your darling isn't moping. Plus, most chocolates contain cocoa which has tryptophan, which in turn helps your body to produce serotonin — the happiness hormone. However, you must keep your eyes open to ensure that none of it gets overdone.

II) Denial During Growing Up Years Could Lead to Binge Eating Later

Gymnastics requires its practitioners to be very light, especially the ladies, but very strong. Remember the Romanian genius Nadia Comaneci who took the world by storm during the Montreal Olympics at the age of 14? She became the first gymnast to score perfect tens — not once, but several times — in her career. From the tender age of seven, she had been denied the joys of living with her family, eating what she wanted to, even normal childhood joys of the occasional bar of chocolate. Eventually, when her performance in the Moscow Olympics was less than impressive, she fell out of public view.

Compensating Childhood Denial

Nadia took to overeating to compensate for denial in childhood and adolescence, eventually being diagnosed with bulimia nervosa. Many people learned that such an eating disorder exists only after hearing about Nadia's condition. Therefore, when you set rules for yourself, or your children, about what to eat, and what not to eat, make sure you don't go overboard about it.

Respect Your Body: You Are a Person, Not a Size

Your body is as unique as you are. Nobody on earth is exactly like you, and no other body on earth is exactly like yours. Respecting your body starts with recognizing all that your body has done for you (and put up with from you!) Remember this is the only one who stays with you from the time you are born to the time of your death. Stop abusing your body with diets, tight clothes, militant exercise, and other self-punishments. Treat your body with dignity — feed it when it is hungry, rest it when it is tired, dress it in comfortable clothes, and move it gently. Just as you rest when you are tired (or, at least should); similarly, listen when your body tells you it is hungry. (Can we?)

III) Unrealistic Standards Make Eating Disorders Flourish

The worst effect of these unrealistic standards is the emergence of eating disorders which are flourishing in this beauty-driven society. Body shaming is so prevalent at every level of society that it has been taking its toll on people, especially the fairer sex, over the past few decades. In India, till the late seventies, a girl or woman was not considered beautiful unless she was comfortably padded. Exposure to international standards of modeling created an aspirational figure amongst women who desired to look like Heidi Klum, Twiggy, Cindy Crawford, or Naomi Campbell. Net result is that these days young girls and women are trapped in a negative cycle of body hatred, which makes them punish their bodies with excessive exercising and starvation. Women with eating disorders are particularly vulnerable to this negative body image cycle. Some go into a flap if they eat a piece of chocolate or dig into a tiny helping of *gajar ka halwa*. That is not the way it is meant to be.

Distorted Body Image Lies at the Root of Eating Disorders

Think of the late Princess Diana who was the heartthrob of millions. In her mind, she, unfortunately, linked her popularity to her body shape and began to suffer from anorexia nervosa. Anorexia nervosa is an irrational fear of being overweight, leading to an eating disorder which makes the sufferers imagine that eating any food will be disastrous for them. This typically makes such people grievously underweight. In the long run, it can give rise to major health issues. Ironically, many young girls who have a naturally skinny figure desire a curvaceous look, and indulge in harmful behaviors to appear more buxom.

IV) Nothing Is More Counter Productive Than a Negative Self-Image

Margo Maine went on to recommend that you "replace the time you spend criticizing your appearance with more positive, satisfying pursuits to let your inner beauty and individuality shine". So, you must understand that a negative body image is a bigger problem than your being too thin, or too fat. You can undo that harm by taking an affirmative stance. Tell yourself that there is more to your personality than your figure. Learn to give your talents, your intellect, and the sweetness of your disposition the credit they deserve.

V) Assigning Yourself Blame for Your Figure or Appearance

Even if you have been so unloving of yourself that you have not taken any care of yourself for years, you should not blame yourself for how you look. Just accept that there is an issue, and you must rectify it proactively. Your appearance should not define how lovable you are, or what respect you should be accorded. You should not stop attending parties, or be terrified of going on vacations because of your figure, or your mental image of what it should be. Accept it if you have any eating disorder (ED), but don't go on a guilt trip over it.

Bolster Your Self-Image

Man, woman, or child, if God created you in a certain way, you should honor that. Tell yourself, "I am fine. I am (trying to be) the best version of me." Don't let others' opinions undermine your self-confidence or your sense of self-worth. In today's society, self-esteem and body-esteem have become one and the same. Unfortunately, this is taking an emotional toll on young girls, and young women. They begin to feel inadequate and often turn to severe behaviors in an attempt to manipulate their bodies to "fit into" an unrealistic standard of beauty. Every time we criticize ourselves we go a level lower, and the groove becomes more permanent.

Make Peace With Your Body Shape

As long as your body shape is not preventing you from doing all that you want to, or creating grave health issues; it is perfect. It is vital that you remain energetic and zestful always. Therefore, if somebody is trying to shame you over a few bonus pounds, or the lack of an ounce of extra fat; put them in their place. We learn to be embarrassed or ashamed of how we feel we look from childhood. You should not be at war with your body, or with what you choose to eat. It is necessary to accept your body as it is for you to be grounded, and then move forward with future plans.

Match Size With Work Profile

If the work you do requires you to stand for hours, the way a doctor or a scientist in a lab might; or to be able to juggle several chores simultaneously — then obviously, you need a sturdier body form than the sylph-like figure that the fashion Nazis expect you to have. Do you imagine that an elfin police woman would be able to physically prevent from wrongdoing, or drag a hefty criminal several yards? Therefore, learn to be practical about what your body size or shape should be.

Cope With the Rigors of Your Profession

A pot-bellied doctor is rare because doctors lead a punishing routine. Doctors need to be trim to be able to cope with the rigors of the profession, and devote their energies to healing patients. However, you need to be aware of the difference between trim and thin. There is a myth that loss of night sleep makes you overweight. In that case, most obstetricians, and many surgeons should have looked like heavyweight champions or Sumo wrestlers. So, you shouldn't allow yourself to strive for impractical proportions. Rather, you should focus on how strong and energetic you are, rather than whether you are elfin or Junoesque.

Don't Let Anyone Dictate What to Eat Or Drink

Take a conscious decision not to force your body to eat or drink what it does not relish, for e.g. boiled food. You should not allow anyone to dictate what you should, and what you shouldn't eat. Reestablish your connection with your body, and feed it what it really needs. A doctor (a topper from London University in the forties) had commented way back in the seventies of the previous century, that most lifestyle ailments occur because we lose touch with our own bodies, and follow regimens which have been prescribed without taking into consideration your specific body type.

Takeaways

- Our feelings often get intricately interwoven with food
- When feeding becomes the panacea for all ills
- Denial during growing up years could lead to binge eating later
- Respect your body: You are a person, not a size
- Unrealistic standards make eating disorders flourish
- Nothing is more counter-productive than a negative self-image
- Bolster your self-image by making peace with your body shape
- Match size with work profile to cope with the rigors of your profession

Chapter 4 — Take Control of Your Life: Put Shame and Guilt Behind You

"It's all fun and games until your jeans don't fit any more." — Anonymous

Raj Kapoor and Rajendra Kumar were excellent friends in personal life. Since they desired to cement this friendship further, Raj Kapoor's daughter Reema was engaged to Kumar Gaurav, Rajendra Kumar's son who was then a star to watch out for. However, after some time the engagement was called off, though the reason was never made public officially. More than a decade later, when Kumar Gaurav had been married to Sunil Dutt's daughter for quite a while, he finally admitted that he called off the engagement because he couldn't watch the way Reema delved into food as though she had been starving.

There Is No Point In Looking Back In Anger, Shame, Or Guilt

There are two major issues here. The first was the judgmental stance taken by the gentleman instead of trying to delve into the root cause or causes. The second is that the lady seems to have used food to deal with her feelings. When binge eating, or overindulgence in comfort food has done its work, there is no point in looking back in anger, shame, or guilt. If people you know, or those whom you don't, indulge in body shaming, you must develop shame resilience. You don't need that zero figure unless you are a fashion model. Be whatever shape you are comfortable with as long as it is compatible with your professional needs.

Shame Is So Universal and So Redundant

Shame is one emotional baggage we would do better to discard as early as possible. Learn to recognize shame as a universal experience, and embrace authentic living as a foundation for shame resilience. When you are expected to conform to certain norms or standards but fall short; the whole process of shaming begins. Body shaming is so prevalent that many don't even realize it when they are being unfairly targeted. Think of all the nasty remarks made when Aishwarya Rai put on weight after her baby. It was as mean as it was unfair. Most importantly, if she was comfortable with her proportions, why were others losing sleep over it?

Body Shaming Is So Prevalent and So Demeaning

It isn't only the film stars, fashion models, and other public figures who are at the receiving end of body shaming. Just about everybody is at the receiving end of such barbs. There will always be that well-meaning aunty or granny who asks whether you don't eat and scolds your mother for not taking care of you, if you are fashionably thin, or have a slight build. Then, there will be the other kind of well-meaning neighbor or relative, who suggests you should take to skipping, or go for morning walks, whether or not your time schedule permits it.

Take Charge of Your Own Body Image

It is your body, and you know what you can do. Just imagine, if Sudha Chandran had listened to the doctors, and given up dancing, we would have lost the art of a great dancer. Instead, she learned how to dance with a Jaipur foot. Suppose Arunima Sinha, who climbed the Everest, had allowed her amputation to deter her from even trying? If you think you can — go ahead. You decide what you want to be like, instead of striving for unrealistic goals. It is more important to realize your dreams and fulfill your aspirations. You should try to ensure that you stay energized to be able to do your duties and follow your hobbies. Trust your inner clock to keep everything in balance.

Think of What You Can Do With Your Body

As Margo Maine's *Body Wars* taught us, we should accept our own body shape as being perfect as it is now. She said, "Think of your body as a tool. Create an inventory of all the things you can do with it." Don't torture yourself with diets, excessive exercise, starvation etc. Find out WHY you added all those pounds, and heal yourself forever by addressing those issues. Think back to a time when you loved the way your body was, and how happy you were to be that way. Get in touch with those feelings again to regenerate a positive self-image.

Practice Critical Awareness

What is the lens through which you view yourself? How do others view you? Or, do you have the self-awareness to perceive yourself with compassion? To be able to do so, use the step suggested by Margo Maine, "Create a list of people you admire who have contributed to your life, your community, or the world. Was their appearance important to their success and accomplishments?" This will serve as a means for you to ground yourself. It will also enable you to veer your energies and efforts from needlessly criticizing yourself, and your appearance.

Gentle Exercise Is the Route to Take

Exercise because it makes you feel good, not to burn calories or shape your body. Forget extreme exercise, grueling routines, and wasting hours on treadmills going nowhere — just get active doing activities you love like walking, biking, hiking, gardening, window shopping, playing with your or your friend's kids/grandkids/pets, etc. When you need to pick up something from the store nearby, walk there instead of taking the car. Dance to a peppy tune. Dance like there is no tomorrow. Most dance forms burn calories, and leave you feeling exhilarated.

Prevent Your Circulation from Becoming Sluggish

Take up some indoor games like badminton, tennis, table tennis. If your job keeps you on desk bound for long hours; keep getting up periodically to walk around. This will ensure that circulation does not become sluggish. Try doing some simple exercises like stretching out your legs under the desk. Getting a massage is good way to improve your circulation naturally. It will also soothe your nerves and tired muscles. Learn deep breathing techniques which will not only calm you, but will also improve the blood circulation in your body. Take up yoga. Quit smoking. Cut back on alcohol which does you more harm than good in the long run. Drink plenty of water. Drinking water periodically reduces hunger pangs too, which is very helpful when following a diet.

Practice High-Intensity Interval Training (HIIT) Only Under Expert Supervision

The person with a lean frame needs more energy to function, than the individual with bonus pounds (and layers of fat). As you work towards converting the fat to muscle, your metabolism begins to speed up. Adding some high-intensity interval training to your regular routine can speed up your metabolism *for the day*. For any long term impact to kick in takes months, if not years, of such training. However, if at any time you feel that instead of energizing you, it is causing aches and pains, stop. HIIT should be practiced only under the supervision of a doctor.

Eliminate temptation: Avoid making a trip to the grocery store when you are upset.

Get emotional support: Call your friend or colleague as this will help you emotionally.

When we get emotional support, our breathing becomes deeper, our heart rate decreases, muscles relax, and we calm down.

Takeaways

- Be whatever shape you are comfortable with as long as it is compatible with your professional needs.
- Shame is so universal and so redundant.
- Body shaming is so prevalent and so demeaning.
- Take charge of your own body image.
- Think of what you can do with your body.
- Practice critical awareness.
- Gentle exercise is the route to take.
- Prevent your circulation from becoming sluggish.

Chapter 5 — HALT Framework to Stop Overeating

"Strange to see how a good dinner and feasting reconciles everybody." — Samuel Pepys

HALT is the acronym for the interlinked emotional and physical states arising out of hunger. Prolonged hunger can cause anger, which has given rise to the word "hangry". Hunger could lead to aggressive behaviour, loneliness, and an overpowering sense of tiredness — the perfect recipe for overeating to compensate for the sense of loss. More than anything else, the sight and smell of food make you run through a gamut of emotions.

H — Hunger Happens to Most People

Hunger occurs when a person is unable to eat at all, or in sufficient quantities to meet nutritional needs for a sustained period. This could be due to dietary restrictions laid out as part of a weight loss regimen, or during treatment of a disease; it could be simply inaccessibility of proper food at your place of work; you might be undergoing training for some sports, when you need to be eating more; or, in case of youngsters, undergoing a growth spurt when your body needs more food. Since hunger and health, even mental health are closely interconnected, it is important to recognize physical hunger, rather than be distracted by emotional hunger. However, here we are not discussing hunger caused by inability to buy food, but by the inability to eat at will.

Constant Hunger Can Be Counterproductive

Patients of chronic diseases like high blood pressure and diabetes must necessarily follow highly restricted diets. This often tends to leave them hungry and angry. Being hungry is stress laden, which makes this hunger in diabetic and hypertensive patients counterproductive. For normally healthy individuals, being occasionally hungry might do them good as it aids in flushing out toxins from the body. When allowing the body to be hungry is overdone, this hunger encourages the body to store food as fat to protect it against probable future "famine". This is often at the bottom of the failure of many diets which rely on making the body starve to convince it to burn stored fat, rather than exercise to burn off excess fat.

Under Eating Might Lead to Overeating Eventually

Being hungry could make it difficult for people to focus, and they might get distracted easily adversely impacting their professional life. For kids and youngsters, it could make them lag in studies. Undereating is just as dangerous as overeating. In fact, research has shown that people who under eat, or have to stay hungry for longer periods, develop food insecurity leading to eventual overeating. The same survey indicated that as many as 30 percent people skip meals when they are stressed.

A — Aggressive/Angry

As indicated above, hunger makes you angry. Unfortunately, there is also the adverse reaction of reaching out to unhealthy food and/or overeating when you are angry. This anger could also result in aggressive behavior when you are ready to take umbrage at the drop of a hat. Such behavior may not necessarily reflect in physical violence; but might show up as raising your voice, threatening people, making rude comments, using abusive language, and displaying hostility towards family members, neighbors, colleagues. The only time anger is justified is when it is directed against social injustice and exploitation of the weaker sections of the society. However, anger caused by hunger hurts everyone, including the person who is angry. Eventually, it leads to a sense of isolation and loneliness. Occasionally, the way to make a person calm down is to offer a glass of water, and some nutritious food.

L — Loneliness

Humans are born to be social. However, the sense of loneliness which besets people after they have indulged in emotional eating and/or overeating is heart wrenching. Not to be confused with solitude which has a calming effect on people; loneliness can be felt even when you are surrounded by people as it creates a sense of isolation. It can adversely impact your ability to solve problems and challenges which assail us daily on the professional front and in our personal relationships. It makes concentrating on any topic difficult; reduces your ability to learn new tricks; take decisions; and encourages negative self-belief. Add to that the burden of weight self-stigma which many people, especially women suffer. It instills in them a sense of worthlessness, shame, and the perception of being discriminated against in social situations due to one's weight. The process of self-stigmatization adversely affects the quality of life, especially the overpowering sense of loneliness that such people suffer.

Reach Out to Your Emotional Support System

This is when you need an emotional support system to deal with your loneliness. It could be friends, family, colleagues, even neighbors who care for you. Just reach out to them. When loneliness keeps growing, it can lead to the structural degeneration of the hippocampus and prefrontal cortex causing depression and anxiety. However, avoid like the plague negative thinking people, and those who are overly critical of everything.

T — Tired

The Stress in America™ survey brought forth many startling responses. Most adults admitted to feeling lazy or simply tired after binge eating, or overeating. After skipping meals due to stress, 24 percent people said that they felt sluggish or lazy, while 22 percent reported being irritable. Millennials are most likely to report feeling sluggish or lazy after skipping a meal (28 percent), compared with 22 percent of Gen Xers, and 20 percent of Boomers. A decrease in energy levels after eating, or feeling of tiredness after a meal is called postprandial somnolence. It is a normal bodily reaction in most people. However, most emotional eaters experience extreme tiredness after they have overeaten, or eaten unhealthy food. Food intolerances and allergies can impact digestion or other bodily functions, and might in result post-meal tiredness.

Get Out of the Rut

Therefore, to help you get out of the rut, and find your food freedom. You must understand the correlation among hunger, anger, loneliness, and tiredness. If a diet keeps you hungry, it is probably harming your body and your mind. Its failure in the long run is almost guaranteed.

Takeaways

- ➢ The sight and smell of food makes you run through a gamut of emotions.
- ➢ Since hunger and health, even mental health are closely interconnected, it is important to recognize physical hunger,

rather than be distracted by emotional hunger.

➢ Hunger makes you angry. Unfortunately, there is also the adverse reaction of reaching out to unhealthy food and/or overeating when you are angry.

➢ Emotional eating and overeating instill a sense of worthlessness, and shame leading to utter loneliness.

➢ Most emotional eaters experience extreme tiredness after they have overeaten, or eaten unhealthy food.

➢ Free yourself from this vicious cycle, and find food freedom under my guidance.

Chapter 6 — Listen to Your Body Signals

"Square box, round pizza, triangle slices, now that's confusing."
— Anonymous

Start eating what you want. Eliminate the concept of good foods and bad foods. Eat what will be satisfying, and will make you FEEL good. Bring back all the foods you've eliminated from your life because somebody, somewhere, at some point said you shouldn't eat them because they had too many calories, too many carbs, too many points, too much fat, or that they just weren't "good for you". The more you restrict the foods you really would prefer to eat, the likelier you are to eventually binge on these same foods (and others).

Demonizing Calories and Sugar

When the editor in chief of a renowned publishing house suddenly passed out in office, everyone from the MD to the accounts personnel went into a flap. It turned out to be hypoglycemia as she ate too little food for her energy needs. Therefore, it is critical for everyone to understand that you need calories for your blood to circulate nutrients and oxygen throughout your body; grow new cells, and repair damaged ones; to even breathe. Your brain needs sugar to regulate your body, generate heat, carry out routine tasks, and even think. If your work entails physical exertion, then you need more calories.

Watch Out for the Empty Calories

What is dangerous for you is the quantum of empty calories you take in — food you eat or drink which lack vital nutrients, but are full of calories such as carbonated cold drinks, packaged fries, and fast foods like pizzas and burgers. Professionals, students preparing for major exams, and mothers of small children rarely have time to sit and eat a leisurely meal. Yet, they are the very people who need to do so more than anyone else. So, they tend to prefer fast foods which are quickly consumed. Empty calories make you feel full quickly, and add to your inches which become twice as difficult to shed. It is no use blaming a sluggish metabolism for those bonus pounds.

Understand the Myths Related to Metabolism

Metabolism is the way your body converts sugar, and other nutrients into energy which is measured in calories, and how quickly or slowly those calories are burnt. Remember that your body shape or size has nothing to do with how fast or slow your metabolism is. Usually, it is determined by genes. With age, your metabolism might slow down, thereby burning fewer calories. The nutrients which aren't burned, are converted into fat, and stored in your body as adipose tissues. Think of how even people like Jackie Chan have gradually added inches over the years despite being a martial arts specialist.

There Are No Moral Issues Involved in Eating

Accept that there is no morality tied to nourishing your body in a certain way, or to enjoying the taste of food. You are not good if you stay on a diet, or bad if you fall off. You are not "better" when you weigh less, or "worse" when you are heavier. The food police might try and tell you otherwise, but your weight, shape, and the way you eat are not, in any way, a reflection of your worth as a person. Yes, it is vital to gain proper nourishment, and in the way you find most attractive.

Trust Your Own Body

Choose today not to play the game anymore. Resolve to learn to eat intuitively — to trust your body to tell you when, how much, and what to eat. Further, if you eat too little throughout the day, your body begins to conserve energy by slowing down the metabolic rate — quite the opposite of the desired result. This is the reason why many diets fail as they depend on fasting. The bigger danger with any diet is that it sets us up for unhealthy habits we can't maintain.

Discover the Satisfaction Factor

Eat what you love. When you let yourself eat what you want to eat, the pleasure you derive will help you feel like you've had enough sooner than if you eat what you think you "should" eat, or are "supposed" to eat. Start by asking yourself what you'd really like to eat — NOT what you "should" eat. Set the table, put out the good china, turn off distractions — make your meals special occasions. Focus on the taste and texture of what you are eating. Enjoy your food, and the whole experience of eating. As humans, we digest really well when we're calm, so we shift into this relaxed state as soon as we start eating.

Challenge the Food Police

Stop the voice in your head (the "food police") that tells you that you are "good" for eating a certain way, and "bad" for eating another way. The food police monitors the collection of rules that you have created as you have gone on and off diets. As soon as you'd like to enjoy a piece of birthday cake or reach for a cookie, you'll hear the food police spit out negative comments, hopeless indictments, and guilt-provoking criticisms. Don't let your food police tell you have no will power, especially if you are under significant stress.

Reject the Diet Mentality

Decide not to diet ever again. Accept the fact that diets are futile. Rebel against the 20+billion dollar diet industry that puts out diet after diet and diet product after diet product while never helping anybody lose weight and keep it off. My eating disorder taught me that I didn't have to be behind bars to experience lack of freedom. I was at war with what I ate and my body. Obesity is one of the nation's fastest-growing and most troubling health problems. Unless you act to address the emotions behind why you overeat, you could be facing long-term problems.

Some Fad Diets

- Atkins Diet used by Jennifer Aniston, and Renee Zellweger.
- South Beach Diet popularized by the Clintons, Kim Cattrall, and Nicole Kidman.
- Mediterranean diet popularized by Penelope Cruz, Brooke Burke, Rachael Ray, and John Goodman.
- Juice cleanse endorsed by Miranda Kerr, and Jessica Alba.
- Vegan Diet used by Natalie Portman, Ariana Grande, Ellen DeGeneres, and Bruce Springsteen.

- Ketogenic Diet endorsed by Rihanna, Kim Kardashian, Halle Berry, and Gwyneth Paltrow.
- Paleo Diet popularized by Jessica Biel, Aaron Rodgers, Jack Osbourne, and Matthew McConaughey.
- The 5-Factor Diet endorsed by Eva Mendes, Lady Gaga, Megan Fox, Rihanna, and Katy Perry.
- Meal replacement shakes endorsed by Kim Kardashian, and Khloe Kardashian.
- The Zone Diet used by Jennifer Anniston, Brad Pitt, Sandra Bullock, Kristen Davis, and Cindy Crawford.
- Detox Teas endorsed by Kylie Jenner, and Khloe Kardashian.
- The Dukan Diet endorsed by Duchess Kate Middleton.
- The 5:2 Diet endorsed by Beyoncé.

Don't Let the Clock Dictate Food Timings

You will notice that the sturdiest babies are those who are demand fed, rather than those who are fed by the clock. You too will be hardier if you follow your body signals. However, the equally dangerous trend is to skip meals because you don't have the time to spend a few minutes to eat a proper meal. Occasionally grabbing a sandwich or burger to allay hunger pangs; don't make it a practice. Your food and drink should contain adequate quantities of fiber, vitamins, micronutrients, and minerals. Further, you should be aware that depriving yourself will only increase your cravings.

Listen to Your Hunger Signals

Few people realize that eating only when hungry is the best way to listen to your body. This will ensure that you eat what your body requires. Too many people are overburdened by what others will think, what the dietician will say, what the fashion police will say. This prevents them from eating the food they desire, and — unless they have shut their ears to their bodies — what they really require.

Respect Your Fullness and Listen for the signs your body sends you when it's satisfied, approaching fullness, and when you are full. After all, you don't follow the clock to go to the bathroom.

Dangers of the Yo-Yo Effect

There is also the risk that as soon as you go off a specific diet, all the lost weight comes rushing back much like the waters of the sea at high tide. This on again and off again weight is a major health threat. You must get to the root cause of this problem and in a lot of cases it is emotional eating. What is likeliest to work for you would be a balanced diet that is formulated of something along the lines of 80% healthy choices, and 20% of simply what you like.

Takeaways

- Eliminate the concept of good foods and bad foods.
- Your brain needs sugar to regulate your body, generate heat, carry out routine tasks, and even think.
- Watch out for the empty calories.
- Metabolism is determined by genes. With age, your metabolism might slow down, thereby burning fewer calories.
- Your weight, shape, and the way you eat are not, in any way, a reflection of your worth as a person.
- Resolve to learn to eat intuitively — to trust your body to tell you when, how much, and what to eat.
- When you let yourself eat what you want to eat, the pleasure you derive will help you feel like you've had enough sooner

than if you eat what you think you "should" eat, or are "supposed" to eat.

➤ Decide not to diet ever again.

➤ Don't let the clock dictate food timings.

Chapter 7 — Manage Internal Chaos of Cortisol

Learnings from Sushant Singh Rajput's Suicide

For many people emotional eating has increased during the lockdown, and working from home as people are assailed by several doubts about their own and their family's future. The stress generated by the pandemic has increased stress levels for many people leading to worrisome levels of depression which has been brought home rudely by Sushant Singh Rajput's suicide.

Consider the Harm Stress Does to Your Body

When we are stressed, it raises the level of cortisol in your body, which demands sugar. So, your body breaks down sugar from the stored fat. While that is good in the short term; in the long run, it can bring in type 2 diabetes, and cause major fat deposits in the belly. The higher the cortisol level in your body, the more alert you are. Conversely, it also becomes that much more difficult to fall asleep. When your body begins to continuously release stress hormones like cortisol, it can result in a wide range of complications, from relationship problems caused by cloudy thinking to significant health consequences, like increased cancer and heart attack risks.

All Of Us Are Hard Wired for Survival

Whatever be the kind of threat we face, or danger we find ourselves in, we fight to survive because all of us are hard wired for survival. As a lawyer had pointed out, even a raving mad individual steps back if he sees a car about to run him down literally. The "fight or flight" reaction we display when faced with imminent danger may be the best-known expression of our survival instinct. This response set is triggered when we perceive a situation as a threat to our existence. Our sympathetic nervous system activates rapid emotional, psychological, and physical changes in response to help us deal with danger more efficiently.

Your Body's Stress Response Helps You Cope with Survival Threats

When your body detects a threat, your autonomic nervous system sounds an alarm telling you something is wrong. The amygdala, an area of the brain involved with emotions, memory, and survival instincts, is activated. Stress hormones which are automatically released, trigger your body's instinctive reaction to danger. This stress response is one of the ways the body helps us to cope with survival threats, but it is helpful only up to a certain point as an extreme response might cause the body to freeze. When catastrophe hits, you are likely to experience some intense emotional, cognitive, and physical stress. Use stress-harnessing strategies — situational awareness, mindfulness, and rehearsal — to increase the chance of surviving an extreme event.

Getting to the Root of the Matter

The instinct for survival is prevalent in all human beings regardless of their sex or age, whether they are rich or poor, highly educated or illiterate. Our brains continually imagine a future that will meet our needs as well as things that could stand in the way of them. Evolution did not simply help us modify our physical being; it also shaped our minds. Evolutionary psychology, in identifying the aspects of human behavior that are inborn and universal, can explain some familiar patterns. It sheds light on why people behave in ways that don't appear to be beneficial to themselves or to their businesses.

Ducking to Avoid Danger Is Ingrained In All of Us

Remember the episode in F.R.I.E.N.D.S in which Joey ducks when Ross tries to hit him, so Ross fractures his thumb? Later, when Joey tries to explain that ducking when someone is going to hit you is a reflex action, Ross stays where he is as Joey demonstrates with a punch to get hit. When you realize the degree of harm emotional eating is causing you, you will try to stop it, and duck the danger by looking for alternative ways to assuage feelings.

Manage stress efficiently: Instead of eating, try some kind of exercise, such as pushups, walking, jogging, weights, or yoga. Try deep breathing or meditating for two minutes. Work on positive self-talk. Use my MYM Framework which I have used very successfully with myself and 1000s of my patients.

Mind Mapping of Emotional Eating Will Throw Up Solutions

It is vital for you to map your mind to understand the underlying triggers of emotional eating. Begin a food journal to record whenever you need to indulge in emotional eating. If you record the feelings you had when you reached for the comfort food, and how you felt afterwards, it will be easier to perform a mind mapping. You should also record timings to help in gaining a perspective as to when you are most susceptible to eating emotionally, especially if you eat to allay feelings of uncertainty or insecurity at a personal or professional level. Frequency will help in indicating how stressed out you are, and how much ground needs to be covered to make you feel in charge of yourself and your life again.

Takeaways

- When we are stressed, it raises the level of cortisol in your body, which demands sugar.
- All of us are hard wired for survival.
- Your body's stress response helps you cope with survival threats.
- The instinct for survival is prevalent in all human beings regardless of their sex or age, whether they are rich or poor, highly educated or illiterate.
- Mind mapping of emotional eating will throw up solutions.

Chapter 8 — 4 Hormones Which Define Your Road to Happiness

"I want to be like a caterpillar. Eat a lot, sleep for a while, and then wake up beautiful." — Anonymous

Happiness is all about how you feel about yourself, the people around you, your circumstances. It stems from the desire to make the very best of your life. Happiness is the secret sauce that can help us be, and do our best. When you are happy, you enjoy better relationships, are less likely to fall ill, and are better equipped to learn new things and acquire new skills. In the long term, happiness makes you feel that you are in charge of your life, emotions, and actions to generate a sense of contentment.

Use the 5-R Framework to Get On Top of Your Emotions

- ❖ Respect — your feelings, and your body
- ❖ Refuel — eat when you need to
- ❖ Rehydrate — keep drinking water
- ❖ Recoup — if you have been ill, rest to recover appropriately
- ❖ Relish — use your five senses when you eat and drink

Release Your Happiness Hormones

Few happy people indulge in emotional eating. So, countering your propensity to eat emotionally by generating your happiness hormones is quite a sensible notion. There are four hormones which determine a human's happiness —

1. Endorphins,

2. Dopamine,

3. Serotonin, and

4. Oxytocin.

We need all four of them to stay happy.

Endorphins: When we exercise, the body releases Endorphins, which helps the body cope with the pain of exercising. We then enjoy exercising because these Endorphins make us happy. Endorphins can also be generated through laughter. Therefore, we should spend 30 minutes exercising every day, read or watch funny stuff to get our day's dose of Endorphins.

Dopamine: Whenever we complete diverse small and big tasks, it releases various levels of Dopamine. It is also released when we get appreciated for our work at the office or at home, making us feel accomplished and good. This also explains why most housewives are unhappy since they rarely get acknowledged or appreciated for their work. Over the years, we buy a car, the latest gadgets, a new house. In each instance, it releases Dopamine and we become happy. So, have you understood why we feel happy when we shop?

Serotonin: Serotonin is released when we act in a way that benefits others. When we transcend ourselves and give back to others or to nature or to the society, it releases Serotonin. Even, providing useful information on the internet like writing information blogs, answering peoples questions on Quora or Facebook groups will generate Serotonin. That is because we will use our precious time to help other people via our answers or articles.

Oxytocin: Finally, there is Oxytocin, which is released when we are close to other human beings. When we hug our friends or family members, Oxytocin is released. The *"Jadoo Ki Jhappi"* from Munnabhai does really work. Similarly, when we shake hands, hold hands, or put our arms around someone's shoulders, varying amounts of Oxytocin are released.

Don't Worry, Be Happy

Therefore, to release Endorphins daily, we should motivate ourselves to exercise, meet up with a friend or friends, the one who get you to smile and laugh. Appreciate others for any small or big help or achievements to release Dopamine. Inculcate the habit of sharing helping others, and reaching out to people in need to generate Serotonin. Most important of all, hug your kids, family, and friends warmly as often as possible to release Oxytocin.

Unlock the Seven Keys to Happiness

You want to lead a life that is free from anxiety, fear, stress, and worry. Don't waste your life being steeped in negative emotions worrying about money, career, relationships. Instead, you should focus on all that is positive in your life. Overall, there are seven essential keys to happiness and success that will help to materialize both in your life.

1 — Gratitude. Be grateful about what you have, your family, your friends, the fact that you have a roof over your head, and food on the table. When you are grateful for your own circumstances, and consider your glass half full, you are less likely to indulge in emotional eating.

2 — Be Present. Transcend the fears of tomorrow and yesterday's regrets to live completely in the present. Problems are a sign of life. Consider them as an opportunity for you to grow as a person, and become more empathetic. Most importantly, while living in the present, don't let your problems destroy your peace of mind.

3 — Manage Time Effectively. Everyone has the same 24 hours to do everything. Efficient time management helps you to achieve more, and waste less time on regrets. Without it, we increase our likelihood for stress, anxiety, fear, and worry to increase chances of emotional eating.

4 — Set SMARTER Goals. When you set SMARTER goals, you're setting specific (S), meaningful (M), achievable (A), relevant (R), and time-based (T) goals that are evaluated (E), and the approach is re-adjusted (R) until you succeed. The more realistic your goals, the better are your chances of achieving them, rather than setting yourself up for disappointment.

5 — Create an Empowering Morning Routine. Keep in mind the old saying, "The morning shows the day." If you want to be happy and successful, create a set of habits in the morning to help foster them in your life. Take control of your life and your routine, grab the reins, be inspired and motivated to achieve something valuable.

6 — Tackle the MITs. The most important tasks (MITs) of the day offer one of the most crucial keys to achieving our goals in life over the long term. Make a list the night before of your MITs that you want to tackle the next day. This will keep you from being overwhelmed as the day progresses.

7 — Focus on Health and Wellbeing. When we do things to harm ourselves by overeating, over-drinking alcohol, taking recreational drugs, and the like, not only does it have an adverse effect on our bodies, but also on our minds. When you are grounded mentally, it helps you incorporate healthy habits into your daily routine without feeling you have been put into a straitjacket.

Takeaways

➤ Use the 5-R framework to get on top of your emotions.

➤ Release your happiness hormones.

➤ Don't worry, be happy by releasing Endorphins daily.

➤ Unlock the seven keys to happiness.

Chapter 9 — Science Behind Habit Formation

"Transform for the better. Age is no bar for that."

Quite often, we do what we do more out of habit, rather than conscious thought. Often, our habits define us — they allow us to survive and function properly in the world. Our brain has been conditioned over the years to react in a specific manner to certain stimuli. Therefore, the brain triggers responses even before we are able to process cognitively what is happening.

This is why habit is called a conditioned reflex action.

Our Brains Love to Create a Routine

Habits are found in an area of your brain called the basal ganglia. The more often you perform an action or behave a certain way, the more it gets physically wired into your brain. Every time you act in the same way, a specific neuronal pattern is stimulated, and becomes strengthened in your brain. Most of what we think, how we react, what we say is guided by habit, which makes us act in a specific way even before our brain has processed the situation. Our brains love automating a sequence of steps to create routine — it saves space for all the other important decision-making processes.

Changing Habits Holds the Key to Stop Eating Emotionally

Habits sometimes need to be changed as they grow stronger over time, and actions or reactions stemming from habit become more automatic. If a habit is hurting you, then it certainly needs to be changed. It is self-defeating if you take the attitude, "If nobody saw you eating, it didn't contain calories." Habits are so powerful because they create neurological cravings: A certain behavior is rewarded by the release of "pleasure" chemicals in the brain. No one should have to suffer the emotional and physical consequences of binge or emotional eating. It means that you begin with not blaming yourself for everything that goes wrong in the world. An effective way to change a habit is to diagnose and retain the old cue and reward, and try to change only the routine.

Our Habits Are Part Of Who We Are

How happy or otherwise you are usually result from the kinds of habits you have. Habit refers to a process whereby contexts automatically prompt action, through activation of mental context-action associations learned through prior performances. Repetition holds the key to habit formation, and to changing it. Remember the connection established by the dictum: watch your thoughts because your thoughts become your words. Watch your words because they become your actions. Watch your actions because they become your habits. Watch your habits because they become your character, and you might be judged unkindly, even unfairly because of certain habits you have. Therefore, the trick lies in breaking free from habits which are crippling your physical and mental health.

Both Breaking and Acquiring a New Habit Are Time Consuming

Whether you're trying to quit a bad habit or institute a new one, it is going to take time. Don't get discouraged if it doesn't happen right away. While it take at least 66 days to form a new habit; it can take only 21 days to change a set habit demonstrating that it is easier to break than to build. So, when you are trying to break the cycle of emotional eating and the guilt trip afterwards — be patient. Focus on the positive changes you are making in your eating habits, and give yourself credit for making changes that will lead to better health.

Keep a Food Journal/Habit Tracker to Stay Consistent

Keeping a food journal will help you identify your food insecurities, as well as the triggers which make you binge on your comfort food. Note what you eat, how much you eat, when you eat, how you are feeling when you eat, and how hungry you are. Over time, you begin to see patterns that reveal the connection between mood and food. In the long run, it will help you practice portion control once you begin noting when you have had even a biscuit. If you get a sense of deprivation when on a diet; it might actually increase food cravings.

Conflicting Messages from the Food and Healthcare Industries

Unfortunately, every person keeps receiving conflicting cues and triggers as the food industry says, health hardly matters, while the healthcare industry discounts the value of healthy eating. The trick is to eat satisfying amounts of healthier foods, enjoy an occasional treat, and get plenty of variety to help curb cravings. Ironically, the worst health impact of emotional eating on your body is that the lack of micronutrients in your comfort food makes you both overweight and malnourished. Given the costs of treating such issues makes healthy eating cheaper by comparison.

Takeaways

- The brain triggers responses even before we are able to process cognitively what is happening.
- Our brains love automating a sequence of steps to create routine.
- The trick lies in breaking free from habits which are crippling your physical and mental health.
- Changing habits holds the key to stop eating emotionally.

- Repetition holds the key to habit formation, and to changing it.
- Keep a food journal/habit tracker to stay consistent.

Chapter 10 - Eating Mindfully

> *"My favorite exercise is a cross between a lunge and a crunch ... I call it lunch."* — Anonymous

In all this, it becomes critical to eat mindfully. Be aware of what is on your plate. The biggest mistake anyone could do is to be watching TV, reading something, working out crosswords in the day's paper, or be on your phone while eating. Gather yourself in to concentrate on what you are eating, chew carefully, and eat slowly. It takes your body about 20 minutes to signal that you are full. Therefore, even if you are simply snacking to bridge the gap between lunch and dinner, and prevent extreme swings in hunger and fullness; do it in moderation.

Eat Rainbow All Three Times to Have a Balanced Meal

Adding color to your food not only makes it look enticing; you add many vital nutrients like vitamins, minerals, iron, carbohydrates, proteins, and fats. You have numerous choices to add color to your meals through salads, desserts, smoothies, shakes, and juices. Non-citrus fruits like bananas, watermelons, papayas, cucumbers, tomatoes, mangoes, pears, coconuts, guavas, kiwis, blueberries, strawberries, peaches, blackberries, raspberries, pineapples, pomegranates, and apples are as delicious as they are nutritive. People who need to avoid sour foodstuffs would do well to add at least some of these fruits to their daily diet.

Make the Most of Your Choices

Not only can you get your daily requirement of Vitamin C from citrus fruits like sweet limes, olives, cranberries, persimmons, oranges, lemons, grapes, avocados, tangerines, Indian gooseberry, grapefruits, mandarins, and cherries; they provide that necessary dash of color to your life. Use all kinds of green leafy vegetables with carrots, pumpkins, cauliflowers, brinjals, beets with potatoes, boiled unpolished rice, bread made from unprocessed flour (without smothering it with butter), oatmeal, *ragi*, millets, *dalia*, and maize to give you the kind of nutrition you need without compromising on taste. Avoid refined flours and polished rice.

Use All Five Senses While Eating

Mindful eating requires you to use all five senses when you have food and drink. Sight, smell, feel (texture), taste, and hearing affect how we react to food. Your meal, or snack should *look* appetizing. You should *want* to eat as soon as you see your food. Typical Mughlai cooking depends significantly on how fragrant it is, and uses spices with an eye to their medicinal properties too. Since the gravy is thin, it seems to be light, but is actually very rich. The Sanskrit expression: *"Ghranen ardha bhojanam"* means that you have eaten half your meal when you have inhaled its fragrance. Every kind of food has its unique texture, which is rarely dictated by the style of cuisine. Whether your food tastes salty, sweet, sour, pungent, or bitter; or incorporates several different tastes to make a complex dish; you will react to the taste in accordance with what your body needs at that moment if you have stayed in touch with your body. The tinkling of crockery often serves as spur to appetite at meal times.

Drink Water Like Food, and Eat Food Like You Are Drinking Water

Water is needed to keep the cells in your body healthy, hydrated, and robust. Drink one glass of water 30 minutes before a meal to help digestion. Remember not to drink too soon before or after a meal as the water will dilute the digestive juices. Drink water an hour after the meal to allow the body to absorb the nutrients. Water aids your body to digest food by breaking it down, and contributes to better absorption of nutrients. It serves to promote the proper function of the enzymes which are secreted in the digestive juices the alimentary canal releases when you eat food. Keeping your body properly hydrated is critical for maintaining good health, and flushing away toxins and free radicals.

Keep Your Body Properly Hydrated

Being hydrated does not refer to how much water you have drunk, but how much water your body is holding at any given time. Suppose you drink two to three liters of water daily, but all of it is being excreted through sweat and urine, then obviously your body is not sufficiently hydrated. It means that you must drink more than that quantity of liquid. Your cells get hydrated when you eat fruits, especially the kind which have a very high water content, like watermelons and oranges. Keep in mind that the starchiest fruits like bananas, avocados, jackfruit, breadfruit, passion fruit are the least hydrating in their natural, freshly picked state. Keep drinking water at short intervals throughout the day to literally wash away the extra acid generated by your body, and maintain the fluid balance in your body.

Partake of Water-Rich Foods That Help You Stay Hydrated

Some foods which help you stay hydrated are peaches, oranges, watermelon, strawberries, cantaloupe, cucumber, skim milk, gourds, and lettuce. Though few people realize it, you are equally like to get dehydrated in winter, when most people drink less water, but have more tea and coffee. Since both tea and coffee have a diuretic impact on your system, drinking them does not rehydrate your body. A better option would be to drink hot, clear soups or broths, which will fill you enough to create a sense of satiety, and nourish you as they usually contain the vital nutrients your body needs. When they have a vegetable, lentil, and/or meat stock as base, you are better served. Throwing in some pieces of vegetables or meat add the necessary crunch that your body needs. When you eat roasted meat, *rotis* or *parathas* made of *maida*, fried food, or very dry vegetable preparations; you should drink plenty of water later to compensate.

Liquid Diets Work When Paired with Sufficient Nutritive Crunch

When you are trying to lose weight, or detox, drinking milk, whey, *lassi*, milk shakes, fruit or vegetable juices, mocktails, and soups are some of the ways you will find the necessary nutrition when you are on a liquid diet. Some rely on protein shakes, but that is not really advisable. It is important to keep in mind that your body needs something to crunch on. Therefore, eat some fresh salad full of fresh vegetables, fruits, and sprouts with minimal or no dressing at some point of the day. If you have a health condition like diabetes, hypertension, rheumatism, or gout, it would be advisable to first seek expert guidance, rather than plunging into the liquid diet. Further, no liquid diet should stretch beyond two weeks.

Listen to Your Body

If your body needs more Vitamin C, as a child you might crave lemons, oranges, and limes. Don't avoid salt, sugar, or even butter if your body is craving them. Many health issues arise because people stop listening to their bodies, and fall into the trap of prescribed menus and timings. Maintain regular intervals between meals without being dictated by the clock. Eating and drinking the right items, while avoiding certain foods and drinks like the plague, will avert many complications in life, including health and weight issues. If you have your food only when your body demands it, the way you drink water only when you are thirsty;

you will achieve portion control more easily. Eat when you want to, what you want to, and in sufficient quantities to ensure that you get the nutrition you need to function efficiently without compromising on taste.

Takeaways

- Gather yourself in to concentrate on what you are eating, chew carefully, and eat slowly.
- Eat rainbow all three times to have a balanced meal.
- Use all five senses while eating.
- Water is needed to keep the cells in your body healthy, hydrated, and robust.
- Keep Your Body Properly Hydrated to maintain the fluid balance in your body.
- Partake of these Water-Rich Foods That Help You Stay Hydrated.
- Many health issues arise because people stop listening to their bodies, and fall into the trap of prescribed menus and timings.

Chapter 11 — The Fundamentals of Nutrition

"Strength is the capacity to break a chocolate bar into four pieces with your bare hands — and then eat just one of the pieces." — Judith Viorst

Few people are mindful of nutritive properties of the food they stock in the home. It is all to natural to reach for that bar of chocolate, or packet of chips when you are feeling nibblish. Here is what you can do instead.

Use a Little Foresight

Keep some fruit of your preference handy for times you feel munchy. If you prefer it to be crunchy, you could also keep a box of mixed nuts — peanuts, almonds, cashew, walnuts — or some muesli in a drawer of your work station. Reaching for a packet of chips or cookies will be self-defeating. You could also bring some fresh salad for your elevenses, instead of reaching for coffee and cookies, or brownies.

Make Your Salads Crunchy

You can make it crunchy with lightly steamed mushroom slices, broccoli florets, and beetroot; tender baby spinach leaves, lettuce, shredded carrots, diced cucumbers; dried cranberries, or any other berry in season; top with sprouts, and peas; sprinkle black salt, black pepper powder, or thinly sliced green chilies, and drizzle with freshly squeezed lemon juice or orange juice. There are as many variations as you can make since you can add any seasonal fruit of your choice, apples, mangoes, lichees, papaya, pomegranate seeds, chia or flax seeds, roasted sesame seeds, pieces of orange instead of the juice, ginger juliennes, even bits of boiled potatoes if you are not diabetic, or steamed sweet potatoes if you are.

Enjoy Being Full Without Feeling Guilty

These kinds of salads can be extremely nutritive, and yet are delicious. Best of all, they give you a sense of fullness without overloading you with calories. Moreover, if pressure at work makes you miss lunch; then you should eat this kind of snack to prevent loss of energy. Add or subtract vegetables and fruits when making your salad. If you are having the salad instead of lunch, then you could add pieces of tofu, soaked chickpeas, boiled eggs, fish like sardines or tuna, or shredded steamed chicken to ensure you have it all. Avoid or go easy on the salad oil for dressing. The more colorful it is, the more appetizing it will look.

Your Daily Diet Holds the Key to Being Healthy

Hippocrates had advised us more than two millennia ago, "Let food be thy medicine, and medicine be thy food." He had recognized that our daily diet holds the key to being healthy. Dry fruits like dates, figs, peaches, pistachios, apricots, and pears (Bartlett) are not only very tasty to eat individually, and when added to food; but they also provide you with the vitamins, minerals, enzymes, fibers, and oils vital for excellent health. Dry fruits and nuts like cashews, almonds, currants, pistachios, walnuts, dried apricots, and plums are some of the richest energy sources. Therefore, delving into a bowl of dry fruits when you are hungry makes perfect sense.

Keep an Eye on How Well Balanced Your Diet Is

Eating a balanced diet which has it all — proteins, carbohydrates, especially whole grains, fat, micronutrients — is your best bet to ensure that you are healthy and fit, which is more important than being willowy or imposing. Always add nuts to your daily menu. Nuts contain phytosterols, compounds that help lower blood cholesterol, and are full of protein, fiber, vitamins, and minerals like potassium, folate, vitamin E, and magnesium. Eat them raw, pound into a paste to create a base for curries, or roast or fry them, and add to sweet or salty dishes for a richer taste. However, avoid candied pineapples, mangoes, and apples if you need to watch your weight, or are diabetic.

Legume it: Remember that legumes like beans — red kidney beans, white cannellini beans — black eyed peas; diverse kinds of pulses; and lentils are great sources of protein, iron, folate, fiber, zinc, and calcium. However, you should remember to first soak beans , chick peas (*Kabuli chana*), Bengal gram (*kala chana*), pigeon peas (*arhar dal*), and lentils before cooking them, to make them more digestible.

Sweet, Sour, Bitter — Eat, Drink, and Be Happy

Even if you have health conditions which compel you to eat or drink some things, or eliminate them from your menu; usually, there are ways of getting round such limitations. Consider a vegetable like radish which many people eat raw as part of their salad, or make parathas with. Few people realize the health benefits of radishes. Just one serving of red radishes provides you with all the vitamins and minerals essential for your diet — a third of your daily vitamin C requirements, magnesium, calcium, potassium, and even zinc. White radish is a good source of vitamin B6, folate, calcium, magnesium, and phosphorus, apart from dietary fiber, vitamin C, iron, potassium, and copper.

Swallowing the Bitter Pill, Or Piling Into a Tasty Dish?

If you have been advised to have bitter gourd to improve your liver's health, or to reduce blood sugar levels, there is no need for you to only drink its juice. Cut the bitter gourd into thin roundels, apply salt and turmeric to them, and crisply fry (ideally using an air fryer) them to eat just like chips, or eat them with roti or rice. There are several delicious recipes through which you can incorporate different kinds of bitter vegetables like bitter gourd, neem leaves, kale, and mustard greens in your meals.

Slake Your Thirst, And Improve Your Health Too

If it is sweltering outside, reaching for a cold drink is alright. Just avoid those carbonated, oversweet cold drinks. You can have a fruit juice of your choice — if it is freshly squeezed, so much the better. Your choices include:

- Milk shakes,
- Iced lemon tea,
- Cold coffee,
- Freshly crushed sugar cane juice,
- Homemade sherbets, especially drinks like *aam panna*,
- Fresh lime juice,
- *Lassi*,
- *Chhaachh*, and
- *Jal jeera*.

Summer or winter, certain vegetable juices work wonders for your health. One such juice which can be drunk even by people who are diabetic combines carrot, Indian gooseberry (*amla*), a finger of ginger, mint leaves, one fresh lime, and a pinch of black salt to make a yummy drink which boosts your immunity. However, don't forget that drinking plain water is the best way to slake your thirst.

Have Antioxidants to Fight Illness

Greens like kale, asparagus, and spinach; vegetables like sweet potatoes, beans, especially red kidney beans, and artichokes; fruits like blackberries, plums, blueberries, and cranberries; and dark chocolate are very rich in antioxidants.

Takeaways

- Use a little foresight when arranging snacks.
- Make your salads crunchy.
- Enjoy being full without feeling guilty.
- Your daily diet holds the key to being healthy.
- Keep an eye on how well balanced your diet is.

- Sweet, sour, bitter — eat, drink, and be happy.
- Swallowing the bitter pill, or piling into a tasty dish?
- Slake your thirst, and improve your health too.
- Have antioxidants to fight illness.

Chapter 12 — You Can Work to Your Full Potential from Today

"Think big and don't listen to people who tell you it can't be done. Life's too short to think small." — Tim Ferriss

You are the only person who can truly decide what you can — and what you cannot — be or do. Only you know what you are really capable of. If you are assailed by doubts, as well you might be; take stock of your current situation, and what you must do to reach your full potential. Think of where you stand in your professional and personal life, and where you want to see yourself. It is your choice when you decide to be the best version of yourself. That is the honorable thing to do. Begin with the premise that you are capable of doing far more than you think. Fear and self-doubt are the greatest enemies of achievement. You can do great work if you tap into your full potential, and are not afraid of achieving your goals.

Throw Off the Burden of the Past to Liberate Your Future

Far too many people carry around the baggage of their past — failures, negative experiences, slights — which hobbles them as they keep harping on what has gone by. Happy or sad, put the past behind you to create the kind of golden future you want to build. If you have been an emotional eater, then put that behind you. Find your food freedom, and transform yourself into the achiever you are. You should not allow yourself to be swayed by what others are doing, and/or their biases. Reward yourself for your successes. It will keep you motivated, and keep the standard of your work high. Once you have a grip on your strengths and weaknesses, your next challenge is to figure out what you truly enjoy doing.

Start Every New Day on a Positive Note

Give yourself some positive reinforcements by telling yourself all that you are capable of achieving, and how you must do so. Start your day right, get up early enough to have a healthy breakfast, leave for work with enough time so you won't be late because of traffic. Plan your activities for the next day at night to ensure that you have your day mapped out. However, you should always allow for a margin of error to ensure that you don't go into a flap everytime a schedule is thrown off due to circumstances beyond your control.

Stretch Yourself to Your Limits

Just as someone else can't breathe for you, somebody else should not set your goals for you, be they professional ones, or personal ones. Don't just think about what is "realistic." The problem with realistic thinking is that it's usually based on what others think is possible. Other people don't know your potential. Whenever you begin a task with a mind towards achieving a specific potential outcome, limit your actions to only those that are required to accomplish that goal. Remember, you won't be able to reach your full potential by holding on to where you are now. Follow the dictum: If it is worth doing, it is worth doing excellently. Make excellence your prime goal, and let the rest flow from there. If need be, acquire new skills, and upskill current ones.

Stay Focused, Be Persistent

It is vital that you don't get distracted from your main goals. You should be disciplined about achieving your goals. Others will criticize you, discourage you by saying that you won't be able to do something or about the difficulties down the road. However, getting good feedback will motivate you, and constructive feedback will make the next thing you do even better. Make sure to ask for feedback from people who are in the know, and who don't suffer from the cockroach mentality. Doing the right thing is a reward in itself — psychologically in the short run, and professionally in the longer run.

Keep Your Eyes Open to New Opportunities

There will always be unforeseen events, or roadblocks which you had not known might exist. Don't let yourself be derailed, and quit. Begin again with renewed vigor. When you treat every new challenge as an opportunity, you widen your scope for improvement. The key to unlocking your potential is continuous effort. You win only when you think you can. Playing safe might prove counterproductive as it would make you hit a plateau. There is nothing anyone can do to prevent you from reaching your potential. The challenge is for you to identify your dream, develop the skills to get there, and exhibit character and leadership needed to get there.

"There is no paycheck that can equal the feeling of contentment that comes from being the person you are meant to be." — Oprah Winfrey

Takeaways

- ➢ Only you know what you are really capable of.
- ➢ Fear and self-doubt are the greatest enemies of achievement.
- ➢ Throw off the burden of the past to liberate your future.
- ➢ Find your food freedom, and transform yourself into the achiever you are.
- ➢ Start every new day on a positive note.
- ➢ Stretch yourself to your limits.
- ➢ Don't get distracted from your main goals.
- ➢ Keep your eyes open to new opportunities.

www.ingramcontent.com/pod-product-compliance
Lightning Source LLC
Chambersburg PA
CBHW070257220526
45465CB00004B/1638